KIDNEY DIALYSIS DIET FOR

BEGINNERS

Recipes that are both delicious and dialysis-friendly

Dr Lily Morgan

COPYRIGHT PAGE

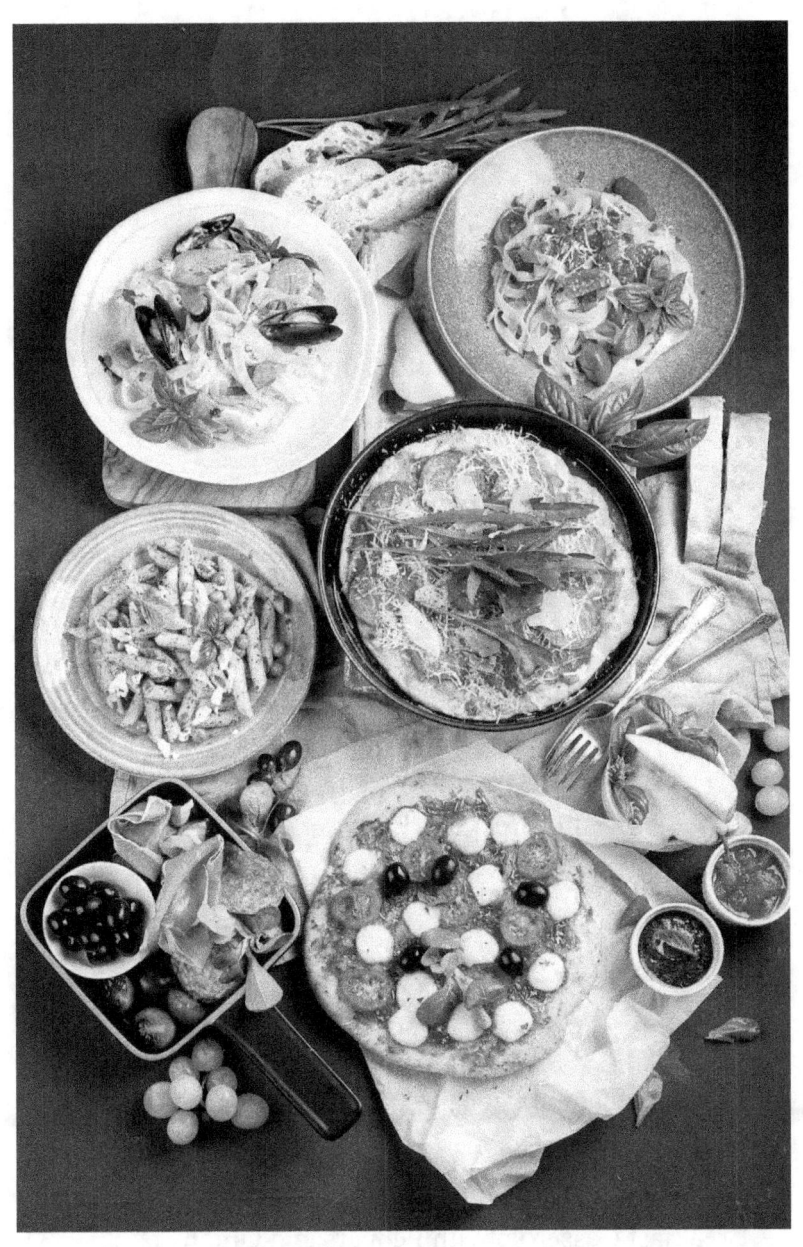

TABLE OF CONTENTS

INTRODUCTION

I n the realm of healthcare and well-being, certain medical conditions require specialized diets to support the management and treatment of the underlying issues. One such condition is kidney dialysis, a procedure used to filter and cleanse the blood when the kidneys fail to perform their essential functions adequately. As the kidneys play a crucial role in filtering waste, excess minerals, and fluids from the bloodstream, their impaired function can lead to the accumulation of harmful substances in the body, potentially causing severe health complications.

The Kidney Dialysis Diet, often known as the Renal Diet, is specifically designed to address the unique dietary needs of individuals undergoing dialysis treatment. This diet aims to optimize kidney function and manage various aspects of the condition, such as fluid and mineral balance, while also promoting overall health and well-being.

Understanding the Kidney Dialysis Diet

The Kidney Dialysis Diet primarily focuses on controlling the intake of certain nutrients to alleviate stress on the kidneys and reduce the buildup of waste products. These nutrients include potassium, phosphorus, sodium, and fluids. By managing the levels of these elements in the diet, patients can better regulate their body's internal environment and enhance the effectiveness of dialysis treatments.

Importance of Following a Dialysis Diet

Following the Kidney Dialysis Diet is essential for individuals undergoing dialysis as it can have a direct impact on their overall health and quality of life. Adhering to the dietary guidelines helps minimize complications associated with kidney failure, such as hypertension, electrolyte imbalances, bone disorders, and cardiovascular issues. Additionally, the diet aids in reducing the workload on the kidneys, which can ultimately contribute to preserving their remaining function.

Guidelines for a Successful Kidney Dialysis Diet

To achieve success with the Kidney Dialysis Diet, it is crucial to have a comprehensive understanding of the dietary restrictions and allowances. A well-balanced diet that meets individual nutritional needs while adhering to the prescribed limitations is the key to maintaining optimal health. Some general guidelines to keep in mind include:

Monitoring Nutrient Intake: Regularly tracking and managing the intake of nutrients such as potassium, phosphorus, sodium, and protein is critical. This often involves working closely with a registered dietitian to create personalized meal plans tailored to the individual's needs.

Protein Consumption: Adequate protein intake is essential for maintaining muscle mass and supporting overall health. However, excessive protein intake can lead to the buildup of waste products, placing additional strain on the kidneys. Finding the right balance is vital.

Fluid Restriction: Individuals with kidney failure may experience difficulty in eliminating excess fluids, leading to fluid retention and edema. Controlling fluid intake is necessary to prevent these complications.

Potassium Management: High potassium levels can disrupt the heart's rhythm, leading to potential cardiac issues. Limiting potassium-rich foods is crucial for maintaining proper heart function.

Phosphorus Control: Elevated phosphorus levels can weaken bones and lead to other health problems. Managing phosphorus intake is essential for preserving bone health.

Sodium Reduction: Lowering sodium intake helps manage blood pressure and reduce the risk of fluid retention.

Nutritional Supplements: Sometimes, dialysis patients may require vitamin and mineral supplements to compensate for the nutrients they cannot obtain adequately from their restricted diet.

Lifestyle Modifications: Alongside dietary changes, adopting a healthy lifestyle that includes regular exercise and refraining from smoking can further support kidney health.

By incorporating these guidelines into their daily routine, individuals can take an active role in managing their condition and promoting better overall health. However, it is crucial to remember that each person's dietary requirements may vary, and consulting with a healthcare professional or registered dietitian is essential to develop a personalized kidney dialysis diet plan.

In the next chapter, we will delve into a comprehensive 30-day meal plan specifically curated for beginners embarking on the Kidney Dialysis Diet. This meal plan will provide a diverse range of nutritious and delicious recipes that adhere to the dietary guidelines while ensuring a well-balanced and enjoyable culinary experience. With the right knowledge and support, individuals can embrace this new dietary journey and foster improved well-being and vitality in the face of kidney dialysis.

Chapter 1: 30 Day Meal Plan

Week 1

Day 1:

Breakfast: Low-Potassium Breakfast Burrito

Lunch: Grilled Chicken and Quinoa Salad

Dinner: Baked Chicken Breast with Asparagus

Snack: Hummus with Carrot and Cucumber Sticks

Dessert: Baked Apples with Cinnamon

Day 2:

Breakfast: Renal-Friendly Oatmeal with Berries

Lunch: Vegetable and Lentil Soup

Dinner: Beef Stir-Fry with Broccoli and Snow Peas

Snack: Guacamole with Baked Tortilla Chips

Dessert: Banana and Strawberry Popsicles

Day 3:

Breakfast: Scrambled Eggs with Spinach and Feta

Lunch: Turkey Wrap with Avocado and Lettuce

Dinner: Lemon Herb Tilapia with Brown Rice

Snack: Greek Yogurt Dip with Pita Bread

Dessert: Chocolate Chia Seed Pudding

Day 4:

Breakfast: Yogurt Parfait with Nuts and Seeds

Lunch: Tuna Salad with Greek Yogurt Dressing

Dinner: Grilled Pork Chops with Zucchini Noodles

Snack: Sliced Apples with Almond Butter

Dessert: Lemon Ricotta Cake (Low-Phosphorus)

Day 5:

Breakfast: Apple Cinnamon Pancakes (Low-Phosphorus)

Lunch: Baked Salmon with Roasted Vegetables

Dinner: Vegetable Curry with Basmati Rice

Snack: Rice Cakes with Cottage Cheese and Berries

Dessert: Vanilla Yogurt with Fresh Berries

Day 6:

Breakfast: Chia Seed Pudding with Fresh Fruits

Lunch: Eggplant and Mozzarella Sandwich

Dinner: Spaghetti Squash with Marinara Sauce

Snack: Cheese and Grape Skewers

Dessert: Poached Pears in Red Wine

Day 7:

Breakfast: Breakfast Casserole with Peppers and Onions

Lunch: Quinoa Stuffed Bell Peppers

Dinner: Stuffed Bell Peppers with Ground Turkey

Snack: Popcorn with Herbs and Olive Oil

Dessert: Watermelon Sorbet (Low-Potassium)

Week 2

Day 8:

Breakfast: Smoothie Bowl with Almond Milk and Banana

Lunch: Black Bean and Corn Salad

Dinner: Egg Fried Rice with Mixed Vegetables

Snack: Trail Mix with Nuts and Dried Fruits

Dessert: Pineapple Coconut Ice Cream (Low-Sodium)

Day 9:

Breakfast: Blueberry Almond Muffins (Low-Sodium)

Lunch: Shrimp and Avocado Salad

Dinner: Baked Cod with Lemon and Herbs

Snack: Celery Sticks with Peanut Butter

Dessert: Berry Parfait with Whipped Cream

Day 10:

Breakfast: Veggie and Cheese Omelette

Lunch: Cucumber and Chickpea Salad

Dinner: Ratatouille with Quinoa

Snack: Veggie Spring Rolls with Dipping Sauce

Dessert: Almond Flour Brownies

Day 11:

Breakfast: Low-Potassium Breakfast Burrito

Lunch: Grilled Chicken and Quinoa Salad

Dinner: Baked Chicken Breast with Asparagus

Snack: Hummus with Carrot and Cucumber Sticks

Dessert: Baked Apples with Cinnamon

Day 12:

Breakfast: Renal-Friendly Oatmeal with Berries

Lunch: Vegetable and Lentil Soup

Dinner: Beef Stir-Fry with Broccoli and Snow Peas

Snack: Guacamole with Baked Tortilla Chips

Dessert: Banana and Strawberry Popsicles

Day 13:

Breakfast: Veggie and Cheese Omelette

Lunch: Shrimp and Avocado Salad

Dinner: Egg Fried Rice with Mixed Vegetables

Snack: Trail Mix with Nuts and Dried Fruits

Dessert: Pineapple Coconut Ice Cream (Low-Sodium)

Day 14:

Breakfast: Low-Potassium Breakfast Burrito

Lunch: Cucumber and Chickpea Salad

Dinner: Baked Cod with Lemon and Herbs

Snack: Celery Sticks with Peanut Butter

Dessert: Berry Parfait with Whipped Cream

Week 3

Day 15:

Breakfast: Renal-Friendly Oatmeal with Berries

Lunch: Grilled Chicken and Quinoa Salad

Dinner: Ratatouille with Quinoa

Snack: Hummus with Carrot and Cucumber Sticks

Dessert: Almond Flour Brownies

Day 16:

Breakfast: Scrambled Eggs with Spinach and Feta

Lunch: Vegetable and Lentil Soup

Dinner: Lemon Herb Tilapia with Brown Rice

Snack: Guacamole with Baked Tortilla Chips

Dessert: Banana and Strawberry Popsicles

Day 17:

Breakfast: Yogurt Parfait with Nuts and Seeds

Lunch: Turkey Wrap with Avocado and Lettuce

Dinner: Grilled Pork Chops with Zucchini Noodles

Snack: Sliced Apples with Almond Butter

Dessert: Lemon Ricotta Cake (Low-Phosphorus)

Day 18:

Breakfast: Apple Cinnamon Pancakes (Low-Phosphorus)

Lunch: Baked Salmon with Roasted Vegetables

Dinner: Vegetable Curry with Basmati Rice

Snack: Rice Cakes with Cottage Cheese and Berries

Dessert: Vanilla Yogurt with Fresh Berries

Day 19:

Breakfast: Chia Seed Pudding with Fresh Fruits

Lunch: Eggplant and Mozzarella Sandwich

Dinner: Spaghetti Squash with Marinara Sauce

Snack: Cheese and Grape Skewers

Dessert: Poached Pears in Red Wine

Day 20:

Breakfast: Breakfast Casserole with Peppers and Onions

Lunch: Quinoa Stuffed Bell Peppers

Dinner: Stuffed Bell Peppers with Ground Turkey

Snack: Popcorn with Herbs and Olive Oil

Dessert: Watermelon Sorbet (Low-Potassium)

Day 21:

Breakfast: Veggie and Cheese Omelette

Lunch: Shrimp and Avocado Salad

Dinner: Egg Fried Rice with Mixed Vegetables

Snack: Trail Mix with Nuts and Dried Fruits

Dessert: Pineapple Coconut Ice Cream (Low-Sodium)

Week 4

Day 22:

Breakfast: Low-Potassium Breakfast Burrito

Lunch: Cucumber and Chickpea Salad

Dinner: Baked Cod with Lemon and Herbs

Snack: Celery Sticks with Peanut Butter

Dessert: Berry Parfait with Whipped Cream

Day 23:

Breakfast: Renal-Friendly Oatmeal with Berries

Lunch: Grilled Chicken and Quinoa Salad

Dinner: Ratatouille with Quinoa

Snack: Hummus with Carrot and Cucumber Sticks

Dessert: Almond Flour Brownies

Day 24:

Breakfast: Scrambled Eggs with Spinach and Feta

Lunch: Vegetable and Lentil Soup

Dinner: Lemon Herb Tilapia with Brown Rice

Snack: Guacamole with Baked Tortilla Chips

Dessert: Banana and Strawberry Popsicles

Day 25:

Breakfast: Yogurt Parfait with Nuts and Seeds

Lunch: Turkey Wrap with Avocado and Lettuce

Dinner: Grilled Pork Chops with Zucchini Noodles

Snack: Sliced Apples with Almond Butter

Dessert: Lemon Ricotta Cake (Low-Phosphorus)

Day 26:

Breakfast: Apple Cinnamon Pancakes (Low-Phosphorus)

Lunch: Baked Salmon with Roasted Vegetables

Dinner: Vegetable Curry with Basmati Rice

Snack: Rice Cakes with Cottage Cheese and Berries

Dessert: Vanilla Yogurt with Fresh Berries

Day 27:

Breakfast: Chia Seed Pudding with Fresh Fruits

Lunch: Eggplant and Mozzarella Sandwich

Dinner: Spaghetti Squash with Marinara Sauce

Snack: Cheese and Grape Skewers

Dessert: Poached Pears in Red Wine

Day 28:

Breakfast: Breakfast Casserole with Peppers and Onions

Lunch: Quinoa Stuffed Bell Peppers

Dinner: Stuffed Bell Peppers with Ground Turkey

Snack: Popcorn with Herbs and Olive Oil

Dessert: Watermelon Sorbet (Low-Potassium)

Day 29:

Breakfast: Veggie and Cheese Omelette

Lunch: Shrimp and Avocado Salad

Dinner: Egg Fried Rice with Mixed Vegetables

Snack: Trail Mix with Nuts and Dried Fruits

Dessert: Pineapple Coconut Ice Cream (Low-Sodium)

Day 30:

Breakfast: Low-Potassium Breakfast Burrito

Lunch: Cucumber and Chickpea Salad

Dinner: Baked Cod with Lemon and Herbs

Snack: Celery Sticks with Peanut Butter

Dessert: Berry Parfait with Whipped Cream

Chapter 2: Breakfast Recipes

In this chapter, we present delicious and nourishing breakfast recipes designed specifically for those with kidney health in mind. Each recipe incorporates ingredients that are low in potassium, low in phosphorus, and low in sodium, making them suitable for a renal-friendly diet.

Low-Potassium Breakfast Burrito

Ingredients:

- 1 whole wheat tortilla
- 1/2 cup egg whites
- 1/4 cup diced tomatoes
- 1/4 cup diced green bell peppers
- 1/4 cup diced onions
- 2 tablespoons low-potassium salsa
- 1/4 avocado, sliced
- Salt and pepper to taste

Instructions:

1. In a non-stick pan over medium heat, sauté the diced onions and green bell peppers until softened.
2. Add the egg whites to the pan and scramble them with the vegetables until fully cooked.
3. Warm the whole wheat tortilla in a separate pan or microwave.
4. Place the scrambled egg whites, diced tomatoes, and avocado slices in the center of the tortilla.
5. Drizzle low-potassium salsa over the filling.
6. Season with salt and pepper to taste.
7. Fold the sides of the tortilla over the filling and roll it up to create the breakfast burrito.

Renal-Friendly Oatmeal with Berries

Ingredients:
- 1/2 cup rolled oats
- 1 cup water
- 1/4 cup fresh berries (blueberries, strawberries, or raspberries)
- 1 tablespoon chopped walnuts
- 1 teaspoon honey (optional)

Instructions:

1. In a saucepan, bring water to a boil, then add the rolled oats.
2. Reduce the heat to low and simmer the oats for 5 minutes or until they reach the desired consistency.
3. Transfer the cooked oats to a serving bowl.
4. Top the oatmeal with fresh berries and chopped walnuts.
5. For added sweetness, drizzle a teaspoon of honey over the oatmeal (optional).

Scrambled Eggs with Spinach and Feta

Ingredients:

- 2 large eggs
- 1 cup fresh spinach leaves
- 2 tablespoons crumbled feta cheese
- 1/4 teaspoon dried oregano
- Salt and pepper to taste
- 1 teaspoon olive oil

Instructions:

1. In a bowl, beat the eggs until well combined.

2. Heat olive oil in a non-stick pan over medium heat.

3. Add the fresh spinach leaves to the pan and sauté until wilted.

4. Pour the beaten eggs into the pan with the spinach.

5. Stir gently until the eggs are cooked to your desired consistency.

6. Sprinkle crumbled feta cheese, dried oregano, salt, and pepper over the scrambled eggs.

7. Serve the delicious scrambled eggs with a side of whole grain toast or a slice of low-sodium bread.

Yogurt Parfait with Nuts and Seeds

Ingredients:

- 1/2 cup plain Greek yogurt (low-sodium)
- 1/4 cup sliced strawberries
- 1/4 cup blueberries
- 1 tablespoon chopped almonds
- 1 tablespoon pumpkin seeds
- 1 teaspoon honey (optional)

Instructions:

1. In a tall glass or parfait dish, layer the plain Greek yogurt, sliced strawberries, and blueberries.
2. Sprinkle chopped almonds and pumpkin seeds on top of the berries.
3. For added sweetness, drizzle a teaspoon of honey over the parfait (optional).
4. Enjoy this refreshing and protein-rich breakfast option.

Apple Cinnamon Pancakes (Low-Phosphorus)

Ingredients:

- 1 cup all-purpose flour
- 1 tablespoon baking powder
- 1/2 teaspoon ground cinnamon
- 1/4 teaspoon salt
- 1 cup unsweetened applesauce
- 1/2 cup milk (low-phosphorus)
- 1 large egg
- 1 tablespoon vegetable oil

- 1 teaspoon vanilla extract

Instructions:

1. In a mixing bowl, combine the all-purpose flour, baking powder, ground cinnamon, and salt.
2. In a separate bowl, whisk together the unsweetened applesauce, low-phosphorus milk, egg, vegetable oil, and vanilla extract.
3. Gradually add the wet ingredients to the dry ingredients, stirring until just combined.
4. Preheat a non-stick griddle or pan over medium heat.
5. Pour 1/4 cup of the pancake batter onto the griddle for each pancake.
6. Cook the pancakes for about 2-3 minutes on each side until they are golden brown.
7. Serve the delicious apple cinnamon pancakes with a dollop of low-sodium whipped cream or a sprinkle of ground cinnamon.

Chia Seed Pudding with Fresh Fruits

Ingredients:

- 1/4 cup chia seeds
- 1 cup low-potassium milk (almond milk or rice milk)
- 1/2 teaspoon vanilla extract
- 1 tablespoon maple syrup (optional)
- 1/4 cup diced mixed fresh fruits (kiwi, mango, and berries)

Instructions:

1. In a bowl, combine the chia seeds, low-potassium milk, vanilla extract, and maple syrup (optional).
2. Stir the mixture well and let it sit for at least 30 minutes or until the chia seeds absorb the liquid and create a pudding-like consistency.
3. Stir the chia seed pudding again before serving to ensure even distribution of the seeds.
4. Top the chia seed pudding with diced mixed fresh fruits for a burst of natural sweetness and flavor.

Breakfast Casserole with Peppers and Onions

Ingredients:

- 4 large eggs
- 1 cup low-sodium cottage cheese
- 1/2 cup diced green bell peppers
- 1/2 cup diced onions
- 1 cup diced cooked chicken (optional)
- 1/4 cup shredded low-sodium cheddar cheese
- Salt and pepper to taste
- 1 teaspoon olive oil

Instructions:

1. Preheat the oven to 375°F (190°C) and grease a baking dish with olive oil.
2. In a mixing bowl, whisk the eggs and low-sodium cottage cheese together until well combined.
3. Stir in the diced green bell peppers, onions, and diced cooked chicken (optional).
4. Season the mixture with salt and pepper to taste.
5. Pour the egg mixture into the greased baking dish.

6. Sprinkle shredded low-sodium cheddar cheese on top.

7. Bake the breakfast casserole in the preheated oven for about 25-30 minutes or until the eggs are fully cooked and the cheese is melted and bubbly.

8. Let the casserole cool slightly before slicing and serving.

Smoothie Bowl with Almond Milk and Banana

Ingredients:

- 1 ripe banana
- 1 cup low-potassium almond milk
- 1/2 cup frozen mixed berries (blueberries, strawberries, and raspberries)
- 1 tablespoon almond butter
- 1 tablespoon chia seeds
- 1 tablespoon shredded coconut
- 1 tablespoon sliced almonds
- Fresh berries and sliced banana for topping

Instructions:

1. In a blender, combine the ripe banana, low-potassium almond milk, frozen mixed berries, and almond butter.
2. Blend the ingredients until smooth and creamy.
3. Pour the smoothie into a bowl.
4. Top the smoothie bowl with chia seeds, shredded coconut, sliced almonds, fresh berries, and sliced banana.
5. Enjoy this nourishing and satisfying breakfast that is packed with antioxidants and essential nutrients.

Blueberry Almond Muffins (Low-Sodium)

Ingredients:

- 1 cup all-purpose flour
- 1/2 cup almond flour
- 1/2 cup granulated sugar
- 2 teaspoons baking powder
- 1/4 teaspoon salt
- 1/2 cup low-sodium milk

- 1/4 cup vegetable oil
- 1 large egg
- 1 teaspoon almond extract
- 1 cup fresh blueberries

Instructions:

1. Preheat the oven to 375°F (190°C) and line a muffin tin with paper liners.
2. In a large mixing bowl, combine the all-purpose flour, almond flour, granulated sugar, baking powder, and salt.
3. In a separate bowl, whisk together the low-sodium milk, vegetable oil, egg, and almond extract.
4. Gradually add the wet ingredients to the dry ingredients, stirring until just combined.
5. Gently fold in the fresh blueberries into the muffin batter.
6. Divide the batter evenly among the lined muffin cups, filling each about two-thirds full.
7. Bake the muffins in the preheated oven for 15-18 minutes or until a toothpick inserted in the center comes out clean.

8. Allow the blueberry almond muffins to cool in the muffin tin for a few minutes before transferring them to a wire rack to cool completely.

Veggie and Cheese Omelette

Ingredients:

- 3 large eggs
- 2 tablespoons low-sodium shredded cheddar cheese
- 1/4 cup diced bell peppers (assorted colors)
- 1/4 cup diced onions
- 1/4 cup sliced mushrooms
- 1/4 cup baby spinach leaves
- Salt and pepper to taste
- 1 teaspoon olive oil

Instructions:

1. In a bowl, beat the eggs until well combined.
2. Heat olive oil in a non-stick pan over medium heat.
3. Add the diced onions and bell peppers to the pan and sauté until softened.

4. Add the sliced mushrooms and baby spinach leaves to the pan and continue to cook until the vegetables are tender.

5. Pour the beaten eggs into the pan over the sautéed vegetables.

6. Cook the omelette until the edges start to set.

7. Sprinkle low-sodium shredded cheddar cheese, salt, and pepper over one half of the omelette.

8. Carefully fold the other half of the omelette over the cheesy side to form a half-moon shape.

9. Continue cooking until the cheese is melted and the omelette is fully cooked.

10. Serve the veggie and cheese omelette with a side of fresh fruit for a satisfying and nutritious breakfast.

Chapter 3: Lunch Recipes

Grilled Chicken and Quinoa Salad

Ingredients:

- 2 boneless, skinless chicken breasts
- 1 cup quinoa, rinsed
- 2 cups mixed salad greens
- 1 cup cherry tomatoes, halved
- 1/2 cucumber, diced
- 1/4 red onion, thinly sliced
- 1/4 cup feta cheese, crumbled
- 2 tablespoons fresh parsley, chopped
- 2 tablespoons olive oil
- 1 tablespoon lemon juice
- 1 clove garlic, minced
- Salt and pepper to taste

Instructions:

1. Preheat the grill to medium-high heat.
2. Season the chicken breasts with salt and pepper. Grill the chicken for about 6-7 minutes per side or

until cooked through. Let it rest for a few minutes before slicing.

3. In a medium saucepan, bring 2 cups of water to a boil. Add the rinsed quinoa and a pinch of salt. Reduce heat, cover, and simmer for about 15 minutes or until the quinoa is cooked and the water is absorbed.

4. In a large bowl, combine the cooked quinoa, mixed salad greens, cherry tomatoes, cucumber, red onion, feta cheese, and chopped parsley.

5. In a small bowl, whisk together the olive oil, lemon juice, minced garlic, salt, and pepper to make the dressing.

6. Add the sliced grilled chicken to the salad and drizzle the dressing over the top. Toss everything together until well combined. Serve immediately and enjoy!

Vegetable and Lentil Soup

Ingredients:

- 1 cup dried lentils, rinsed and drained
- 6 cups vegetable broth

- 1 tablespoon olive oil
- 1 onion, diced
- 2 carrots, diced
- 2 celery stalks, diced
- 2 cloves garlic, minced
- 1 teaspoon ground cumin
- 1 teaspoon ground coriander
- 1/2 teaspoon smoked paprika
- 1 bay leaf
- Salt and pepper to taste
- Fresh parsley for garnish

Instructions:

1. In a large pot, heat the olive oil over medium heat. Add the diced onion, carrots, and celery. Sauté for about 5 minutes or until the vegetables are softened.
2. Add the minced garlic, ground cumin, ground coriander, smoked paprika, bay leaf, salt, and pepper. Stir well to coat the vegetables in the spices.
3. Pour in the vegetable broth and add the rinsed lentils. Bring the soup to a boil, then reduce heat to

low, cover, and let it simmer for about 20-25 minutes or until the lentils are tender.

4. Remove the bay leaf from the soup and adjust seasoning with more salt and pepper if needed.

5. Ladle the vegetable and lentil soup into bowls and garnish with fresh parsley. Serve hot and enjoy this comforting and nutritious soup!

Turkey Wrap with Avocado and Lettuce

Ingredients:

- 4 large whole wheat tortillas or wraps
- 1 pound deli-sliced turkey breast
- 1 ripe avocado, sliced
- 1 cup lettuce leaves
- 1/2 cup cherry tomatoes, halved
- 1/4 cup mayonnaise
- 2 tablespoons Dijon mustard
- Salt and pepper to taste

Instructions:

1. Lay out the whole wheat tortillas on a clean surface.
2. In a small bowl, mix together the mayonnaise and Dijon mustard. Spread this mixture evenly on each tortilla.
3. Divide the deli-sliced turkey breast, avocado slices, lettuce leaves, and cherry tomatoes among the tortillas.
4. Season with salt and pepper to taste.
5. Roll up each tortilla tightly, forming a wrap.
6. Slice the wraps in half diagonally and serve. These turkey wraps are perfect for a quick and delicious lunch on the go!

Tuna Salad with Greek Yogurt Dressing

Ingredients:

- 2 cans tuna, drained
- 1/2 cup plain Greek yogurt
- 1 tablespoon lemon juice
- 1/4 cup diced cucumber
- 1/4 cup diced red bell pepper

- 2 green onions, sliced
- 2 tablespoons fresh dill, chopped
- Salt and pepper to taste
- Lettuce leaves for serving

Instructions:

1. In a medium bowl, combine the drained tuna, Greek yogurt, lemon juice, diced cucumber, diced red bell pepper, sliced green onions, and chopped dill.
2. Mix everything together until well combined.
3. Season the tuna salad with salt and pepper to taste.
4. Serve the tuna salad on a bed of lettuce leaves or as a sandwich filling. Enjoy this protein-packed and flavorful lunch option!

Baked Salmon with Roasted Vegetables

Ingredients:

- 4 salmon fillets
- 2 tablespoons olive oil
- 1 teaspoon dried thyme

- 1 teaspoon dried rosemary
- 1 teaspoon garlic powder
- Salt and pepper to taste
- 1 cup cherry tomatoes
- 1 cup asparagus spears
- 1 cup baby potatoes, halved

Instructions:

1. Preheat the oven to 400°F (200°C) and line a baking sheet with parchment paper.
2. Place the salmon fillets on the prepared baking sheet.
3. In a small bowl, mix together the olive oil, dried thyme, dried rosemary, garlic powder, salt, and pepper.
4. Brush the olive oil mixture over the salmon fillets, making sure they are evenly coated.
5. Arrange the cherry tomatoes, asparagus spears, and halved baby potatoes around the salmon on the baking sheet.
6. Drizzle a little olive oil over the vegetables and season with salt and pepper.

7. Bake in the preheated oven for about 15-20 minutes or until the salmon is cooked through and the vegetables are tender.

8. Serve the baked salmon with roasted vegetables for a healthy and satisfying lunch option!

Eggplant and Mozzarella Sandwich

Ingredients:

- 1 large eggplant, sliced
- 1 cup all-purpose flour
- 2 large eggs, beaten
- 2 cups breadcrumbs
- Salt and pepper to taste
- 4 ciabatta rolls or sandwich buns
- 1 cup marinara sauce
- 8 slices fresh mozzarella cheese
- Fresh basil leaves for garnish

Instructions:

1. Preheat the oven to 400°F (200°C) and line a baking sheet with parchment paper.

2. Season the eggplant slices with salt and pepper.

3. Set up a breading station with three shallow dishes: one with all-purpose flour, one with beaten eggs, and one with breadcrumbs.

4. Dip each eggplant slice into the flour, then the beaten eggs, and finally coat it with breadcrumbs.

5. Place the breaded eggplant slices on the prepared baking sheet.

6. Bake in the preheated oven for about 15-20 minutes or until the eggplant is crispy and golden brown.

7. Slice the ciabatta rolls or sandwich buns in half and spread marinara sauce on each side.

8. Layer the baked eggplant slices and fresh mozzarella cheese on the bottom half of the rolls.

9. Garnish with fresh basil leaves and cover with the top half of the rolls.

10. Serve the eggplant and mozzarella sandwiches warm for a delightful and hearty lunch!

Quinoa Stuffed Bell Peppers

Ingredients:

- 4 large bell peppers, any color
- 1 cup quinoa, rinsed

- 2 cups vegetable broth
- 1 tablespoon olive oil
- 1 onion, diced
- 2 cloves garlic, minced
- 1 zucchini, diced
- 1 cup cherry tomatoes, halved
- 1/2 cup black olives, sliced
- 1/4 cup fresh parsley, chopped
- 1 teaspoon dried oregano
- 1 teaspoon dried basil
- Salt and pepper to taste
- 1/2 cup shredded mozzarella cheese

Instructions:

1. Preheat the oven to 375°F (190°C) and grease a baking dish.
2. Cut the tops off the bell peppers and remove the seeds and membranes from the inside.
3. In a medium saucepan, bring the vegetable broth to a boil. Add the rinsed quinoa, reduce heat, cover, and simmer for about 15 minutes or until the quinoa is cooked and the liquid is absorbed.

4. In a large skillet, heat the olive oil over medium heat. Add the diced onion and minced garlic, sautéing until the onion is translucent.

5. Add the diced zucchini, halved cherry tomatoes, sliced black olives, chopped parsley, dried oregano, dried basil, salt, and pepper to the skillet. Cook for about 5 minutes or until the vegetables are tender.

6. Stir in the cooked quinoa and mix everything together until well combined.

7. Stuff each bell pepper with the quinoa and vegetable mixture, pressing it down gently.

8. Place the stuffed bell peppers in the prepared baking dish and cover with foil.

9. Bake in the preheated oven for about 20 minutes.

10. Remove the foil, sprinkle shredded mozzarella cheese on top of each stuffed bell pepper, and bake for an additional 5 minutes or until the cheese is melted and bubbly.

11. Serve the quinoa stuffed bell peppers as a flavorful and nutritious lunch option!

Black Bean and Corn Salad

Ingredients:

- 2 cups cooked black beans
- 1 cup corn kernels (fresh, frozen, or canned)
- 1 red bell pepper, diced
- 1/4 cup red onion, finely chopped
- 1/4 cup fresh cilantro, chopped
- 1 jalapeno, seeded and minced (optional for heat)
- 2 tablespoons lime juice
- 2 tablespoons olive oil
- 1 teaspoon ground cumin
- Salt and pepper to taste
- Tortilla chips for serving

Instructions:

1. In a large bowl, combine the cooked black beans, corn kernels, diced red bell pepper, finely chopped red onion, chopped cilantro, and minced jalapeno (if using).

2. In a small bowl, whisk together the lime juice, olive oil, ground cumin, salt, and pepper to make the dressing.

3. Pour the dressing over the black bean and corn salad and toss everything together until well coated.

4. Cover the bowl with plastic wrap and refrigerate for at least 30 minutes to allow the flavors to meld.

5. Serve the black bean and corn salad with tortilla chips for a refreshing and satisfying lunch!

Shrimp and Avocado Salad

Ingredients:

- 1 pound large shrimp, peeled and deveined
- 1 tablespoon olive oil
- 1 teaspoon paprika
- 1/2 teaspoon garlic powder
- Salt and pepper to taste
- 4 cups mixed salad greens
- 1 avocado, diced
- 1/2 cup cherry tomatoes, halved
- 1/4 cup red onion, thinly sliced
- 2 tablespoons fresh cilantro, chopped
- 2 tablespoons lime juice
- 2 tablespoons olive oil
- Salt and pepper to taste

Instructions:

1. In a medium bowl, toss the peeled and deveined shrimp with olive oil, paprika, garlic powder, salt, and pepper until well coated.
2. Heat a large skillet over medium-high heat. Add the seasoned shrimp to the skillet and cook for about 2-3 minutes per side or until the shrimp is pink and cooked through.
3. In a large bowl, combine the mixed salad greens, diced avocado, halved cherry tomatoes, thinly sliced red onion, and chopped cilantro.
4. In a small bowl, whisk together the lime juice, olive oil, salt, and pepper to make the dressing.
5. Add the cooked shrimp to the salad and drizzle the dressing over the top. Toss everything together until well combined.
6. Serve the shrimp and avocado salad for a light and flavorful lunch option!

Cucumber and Chickpea Salad

Ingredients:

- 2 cups cooked chickpeas
- 1 cucumber, diced
- 1/2 red bell pepper, diced
- 1/4 cup red onion, finely chopped
- 1/4 cup fresh parsley, chopped
- 1/4 cup fresh mint, chopped
- 2 tablespoons lemon juice
- 2 tablespoons olive oil
- 1 teaspoon ground cumin
- Salt and pepper to taste

Instructions:

1. In a large bowl, combine the cooked chickpeas, diced cucumber, diced red bell pepper, finely chopped red onion, chopped parsley, and chopped mint.
2. In a small bowl, whisk together the lemon juice, olive oil, ground cumin, salt, and pepper to make the dressing.

3. Pour the dressing over the cucumber and chickpea salad and toss everything together until well coated.
4. Cover the bowl with plastic wrap and refrigerate for at least 30 minutes to allow the flavors to meld.
5. Serve the cucumber and chickpea salad as a refreshing and nutritious lunch option!

Chapter 4: Dinner Recipes

In this chapter, we will explore delectable and wholesome dinner recipes that cater to the dietary needs of those on a kidney dialysis diet. Each recipe offers a delightful blend of flavors, nutrition, and easy preparation, making them ideal choices for beginners and seasoned cooks alike.

Baked Chicken Breast with Asparagus

Ingredients:

- 4 boneless, skinless chicken breasts
- 1 bunch of fresh asparagus spears
- 2 tablespoons olive oil
- 2 cloves garlic, minced
- 1 teaspoon dried thyme
- 1 teaspoon dried rosemary
- Salt and pepper to taste

Instructions:

1. Preheat the oven to 375°F (190°C).

2. Rinse the chicken breasts and pat them dry with paper towels. Place them in a baking dish.

3. Trim the tough ends of the asparagus and arrange them around the chicken breasts in the baking dish.

4. Drizzle the olive oil over the chicken and asparagus. Sprinkle minced garlic, dried thyme, dried rosemary, salt, and pepper evenly over the chicken.

5. Cover the baking dish with foil and bake for 25-30 minutes or until the chicken is cooked through and reaches an internal temperature of 165°F (74°C).

6. Remove the foil for the last 5 minutes of baking to allow the chicken to brown slightly.

7. Serve the baked chicken breast with asparagus and enjoy!

Beef Stir-Fry with Broccoli and Snow Peas

Ingredients:
- 1 lb (450g) beef sirloin, thinly sliced
- 2 cups broccoli florets
- 1 cup snow peas

- 1 red bell pepper, sliced
- 3 tablespoons low-sodium soy sauce
- 2 tablespoons oyster sauce
- 1 tablespoon sesame oil
- 2 cloves garlic, minced
- 1-inch piece of ginger, grated
- 2 tablespoons vegetable oil
- Sesame seeds for garnish (optional)

Instructions:

1. In a bowl, mix low-sodium soy sauce, oyster sauce, and sesame oil to create the marinade. Add the sliced beef and let it marinate for at least 20 minutes.
2. Heat vegetable oil in a wok or large skillet over medium-high heat. Add minced garlic and grated ginger, stirring for about 30 seconds until fragrant.
3. Add the marinated beef to the wok and stir-fry for 2-3 minutes until it's browned.
4. Add broccoli florets, snow peas, and sliced red bell pepper to the wok. Continue to stir-fry for an

additional 3-4 minutes until the vegetables are tender-crisp and the beef is cooked to your liking.

5. Serve the beef stir-fry over brown rice or quinoa. Garnish with sesame seeds if desired.

Lemon Herb Tilapia with Brown Rice

Ingredients:

- 4 tilapia fillets
- 2 lemons, sliced
- 2 tablespoons olive oil
- 2 tablespoons fresh parsley, chopped
- 1 tablespoon fresh dill, chopped
- 1 tablespoon fresh thyme, chopped
- 1 teaspoon paprika
- Salt and pepper to taste
- 2 cups cooked brown rice

Instructions:

1. Preheat the oven to 400°F (200°C).
2. Place the tilapia fillets in a baking dish and drizzle olive oil over them. Season with chopped parsley, dill, thyme, paprika, salt, and pepper.

3. Arrange lemon slices on top of each tilapia fillet.

4. Cover the baking dish with foil and bake for 15-20 minutes or until the fish is cooked through and flakes easily with a fork.

5. Serve the lemon herb tilapia over a bed of cooked brown rice and enjoy the flavorful combination.

Grilled Pork Chops with Zucchini Noodles

Ingredients:

- 4 boneless pork chops
- 2 medium zucchinis, spiralized into noodles
- 2 tablespoons olive oil
- 1 teaspoon dried basil
- 1 teaspoon dried oregano
- 1 teaspoon garlic powder
- Salt and pepper to taste

Instructions:

1. Preheat the grill to medium-high heat.

2. Rub the pork chops with olive oil, dried basil, dried oregano, garlic powder, salt, and pepper.

3. Grill the pork chops for about 4-5 minutes on each side or until they reach an internal temperature of 145°F (63°C).

4. While the pork chops are grilling, heat olive oil in a large skillet over medium heat. Add the zucchini noodles and sauté for 2-3 minutes until tender.

5. Serve the grilled pork chops over the zucchini noodles and enjoy this delicious and healthy dinner option.

Vegetable Curry with Basmati Rice

Ingredients:
- 1 cup basmati rice
- 2 cups mixed vegetables (carrots, bell peppers, peas, etc.)
- 1 can (14 oz) diced tomatoes
- 1 can (14 oz) coconut milk
- 1 tablespoon curry powder
- 1 teaspoon cumin
- 1 teaspoon turmeric

- 1 tablespoon vegetable oil
- Salt and pepper to taste
- Fresh cilantro for garnish (optional)

Instructions:

1. Cook basmati rice according to package instructions and set aside.
2. In a large skillet, heat vegetable oil over medium heat. Add curry powder, cumin, turmeric, salt, and pepper. Stir for about 30 seconds until fragrant.
3. Add mixed vegetables to the skillet and sauté for 2-3 minutes until slightly softened.
4. Pour in the diced tomatoes and coconut milk. Stir to combine all the ingredients and let the mixture simmer for 10-12 minutes, allowing the flavors to meld together.
5. Serve the vegetable curry over a bed of basmati rice. Garnish with fresh cilantro if desired.

Spaghetti Squash with Marinara Sauce

Ingredients:

- 1 medium spaghetti squash
- 2 cups low-sodium marinara sauce
- 1 tablespoon olive oil
- 2 cloves garlic, minced
- 1 teaspoon dried basil
- 1 teaspoon dried oregano
- Salt and pepper to taste
- Grated Parmesan cheese for topping (optional)

Instructions:

1. Preheat the oven to 375°F (190°C).
2. Cut the spaghetti squash in half lengthwise and scoop out the seeds and membranes.
3. Place the squash halves, cut side down, in a baking dish. Add a little water to the dish to create steam and cover with foil.
4. Bake the spaghetti squash in the preheated oven for 40-45 minutes or until the flesh is tender and easily comes apart into spaghetti-like strands with a fork.

5. While the squash is baking, prepare the marinara sauce. In a saucepan, heat olive oil over medium heat. Add minced garlic, dried basil, dried oregano, salt, and pepper. Sauté for about 30 seconds until fragrant.

6. Pour the low-sodium marinara sauce into the saucepan and let it simmer for 10-15 minutes, stirring occasionally.

7. Once the spaghetti squash is ready, scrape the flesh with a fork to create spaghetti-like strands. Serve the squash with the marinara sauce on top. Add grated Parmesan cheese as a final touch if desired.

Stuffed Bell Peppers with Ground Turkey

Ingredients:

- 4 large bell peppers (any color), tops removed and seeds removed
- 1 lb (450g) ground turkey
- 1 cup cooked quinoa
- 1 can (14 oz) diced tomatoes

- 1 cup low-sodium vegetable broth
- 1 small onion, diced
- 2 cloves garlic, minced
- 1 teaspoon dried oregano
- 1 teaspoon dried basil
- Salt and pepper to taste
- Shredded mozzarella cheese for topping (optional)

Instructions:

1. Preheat the oven to 375°F (190°C).
2. In a skillet, cook ground turkey over medium heat until it's no longer pink. Drain any excess fat.
3. Add diced onion and minced garlic to the skillet and sauté until they become translucent.
4. Stir in cooked quinoa, diced tomatoes, dried oregano, dried basil, salt, and pepper. Pour in low-sodium vegetable broth and let the mixture simmer for 5-7 minutes, allowing the flavors to meld together.
5. Stuff each bell pepper with the turkey-quinoa mixture and place them in a baking dish.

6. Cover the baking dish with foil and bake the stuffed bell peppers for 25-30 minutes or until the peppers are tender.

7. If desired, sprinkle shredded mozzarella cheese over the top of each stuffed pepper and return to the oven for an additional 5 minutes to melt the cheese.

8. Serve the stuffed bell peppers hot and enjoy this nutritious and flavorful dinner.

Egg Fried Rice with Mixed Vegetables

Ingredients:

- 2 cups cooked brown rice
- 4 large eggs, lightly beaten
- 1 cup mixed vegetables (peas, carrots, corn, etc.)
- 2 tablespoons low-sodium soy sauce
- 1 tablespoon vegetable oil
- 2 green onions, chopped
- 1 teaspoon sesame oil (optional)
- Salt and pepper to taste

Instructions:

1. In a wok or large skillet, heat vegetable oil over medium heat.

2. Add the lightly beaten eggs to the wok and scramble them until they are cooked through. Remove the eggs from the wok and set them aside.

3. In the same wok, add mixed vegetables and sauté for 2-3 minutes until they are tender.

4. Stir in cooked brown rice and scrambled eggs. Drizzle low-sodium soy sauce and sesame oil over the mixture. Toss everything together until well combined.

5. Season with salt and pepper to taste.

6. Garnish the egg fried rice with chopped green onions before serving, and enjoy this quick and satisfying dinner option.

Baked Cod with Lemon and Herbs

Ingredients:

- 4 cod fillets
- 2 lemons, juiced and zested
- 2 tablespoons fresh parsley, chopped

- 1 tablespoon fresh dill, chopped
- 1 tablespoon fresh thyme, chopped
- 2 cloves garlic, minced
- 2 tablespoons olive oil
- Salt and pepper to taste

Instructions:

1. Preheat the oven to 375°F (190°C).
2. Place the cod fillets in a baking dish.
3. In a small bowl, mix the juice and zest of one lemon, chopped parsley, dill, thyme, minced garlic, olive oil, salt, and pepper to create the marinade.
4. Pour the marinade over the cod fillets, making sure they are evenly coated.
5. Slice the second lemon and place the lemon slices on top of each cod fillet.
6. Cover the baking dish with foil and bake for 15-20 minutes or until the cod is cooked through and flakes easily with a fork.
7. Serve the baked cod with lemon and herbs alongside your favorite kidney-friendly side dish and enjoy!

Ratatouille with Quinoa

Ingredients:

- 1 eggplant, diced
- 1 zucchini, diced
- 1 yellow squash, diced
- 1 red bell pepper, diced
- 1 yellow bell pepper, diced
- 1 can (14 oz) diced tomatoes
- 2 tablespoons olive oil
- 2 cloves garlic, minced
- 1 teaspoon dried thyme
- 1 teaspoon dried rosemary
- 1 teaspoon dried oregano
- Salt and pepper to taste
- 2 cups cooked quinoa

Instructions:

1. In a large skillet, heat olive oil over medium heat.
2. Add diced eggplant, zucchini, yellow squash, red bell pepper, and yellow bell pepper to the skillet. Sauté for 5-7 minutes until the vegetables are slightly softened.

3. Stir in minced garlic, dried thyme, dried rosemary, dried oregano, salt, and pepper. Continue to sauté for an additional 2-3 minutes until the vegetables are tender.

4. Pour in the diced tomatoes and let the mixture simmer for 10-12 minutes, allowing the flavors to blend together.

5. Serve the ratatouille over cooked quinoa and enjoy this delightful and hearty dinner option.

Chapter 5: Snacks and Appetizers

In this chapter, we'll explore delectable snacks and appetizers, specially curated to provide you with wholesome goodness and keep your taste buds satisfied.

Hummus with Carrot and Cucumber Sticks

Ingredients:

- 1 can (15 ounces) chickpeas (garbanzo beans), drained and rinsed
- 2 garlic cloves, minced
- 1/4 cup tahini
- 3 tablespoons lemon juice
- 1/4 cup water
- 2 tablespoons olive oil
- 1/2 teaspoon ground cumin
- Salt and pepper to taste
- Carrot sticks and cucumber sticks for dipping

Instructions:

1. In a food processor, combine the chickpeas, minced garlic, tahini, lemon juice, water, olive oil, cumin, salt, and pepper.
2. Blend the mixture until smooth and creamy, adding more water if needed to achieve the desired consistency.
3. Transfer the hummus to a serving bowl and refrigerate for at least 30 minutes to allow the flavors to meld.
4. Serve with carrot and cucumber sticks for a refreshing and nutrient-packed snack.

Guacamole with Baked Tortilla Chips

Ingredients:
- 2 ripe avocados, peeled and pitted
- 1/4 cup diced tomatoes
- 1/4 cup diced onions
- 1 jalapeno, seeded and finely chopped (optional for spice)
- 2 tablespoons chopped fresh cilantro

- 1 lime, juiced
- Salt and pepper to taste
- Baked tortilla chips for serving

Instructions:

1. In a mixing bowl, mash the avocados until smooth, leaving some small chunks for texture.
2. Stir in the diced tomatoes, onions, jalapeno (if using), cilantro, lime juice, salt, and pepper.
3. Mix all the ingredients thoroughly to ensure even distribution of flavors.
4. Cover the bowl with plastic wrap, pressing it against the guacamole's surface to prevent browning, and refrigerate for at least 30 minutes.
5. Serve with baked tortilla chips for a zesty and nutrient-rich appetizer.

Greek Yogurt Dip with Pita Bread

Ingredients:
- 1 cup plain Greek yogurt
- 2 tablespoons chopped fresh dill
- 1 tablespoon chopped fresh mint

- 1 tablespoon lemon juice
- 1 garlic clove, minced
- Salt and pepper to taste
- Whole grain pita bread, cut into triangles, for dipping

Instructions:

1. In a bowl, combine the Greek yogurt, chopped dill, chopped mint, lemon juice, minced garlic, salt, and pepper.
2. Mix well until all the ingredients are thoroughly incorporated.
3. Refrigerate the dip for at least 20 minutes to allow the flavors to meld.
4. Serve with whole grain pita bread triangles for a creamy and flavorful snack.

Sliced Apples with Almond Butter

Ingredients:
- 2 apples, cored and sliced
- 1/4 cup almond butter

Instructions:

1. Arrange the apple slices on a plate or serving tray.

2. Place the almond butter in a small bowl for dipping.

3. Dip the apple slices into the almond butter for a crunchy and protein-rich snack.

Rice Cakes with Cottage Cheese and Berries

Ingredients:

- 2 rice cakes
- 1/2 cup low-fat cottage cheese
- Assorted fresh berries (strawberries, blueberries, raspberries) for topping

Instructions:

1. Spread the low-fat cottage cheese evenly over each rice cake.

2. Top with assorted fresh berries for a delightful and low-sodium treat.

Cheese and Grape Skewers

Ingredients:

- Cubed low-sodium cheese (cheddar, mozzarella, or Swiss)
- Fresh grapes

Instructions:

1. Thread the cubed cheese and fresh grapes alternately onto skewers.
2. Arrange the skewers on a serving platter for an elegant and calcium-rich appetizer.

Popcorn with Herbs and Olive Oil

Ingredients:

- 1/2 cup popcorn kernels
- 2 tablespoons olive oil
- Dried herbs (rosemary, thyme, oregano) for seasoning
- Salt to taste

Instructions:

1. Pop the popcorn kernels using an air popper or stovetop method.
2. Drizzle the olive oil over the popped popcorn and toss to coat evenly.
3. Season with dried herbs and salt for a savory and crunchy snack.

Trail Mix with Nuts and Dried Fruits

Ingredients:
- 1/2 cup unsalted almonds
- 1/2 cup unsalted walnuts
- 1/2 cup unsalted pistachios
- 1/2 cup dried cranberries
- 1/2 cup dried apricots, chopped
- 1/4 cup pumpkin seeds

Instructions:
1. In a large mixing bowl, combine all the ingredients.
2. Toss the mixture to evenly distribute the nuts and dried fruits.
3. Transfer the trail mix to an airtight container for a protein-packed and portable snack.

Celery Sticks with Peanut Butter

Ingredients:

- Celery sticks
- Natural peanut butter

Instructions:

1. Fill the celery sticks with natural peanut butter for a crunchy and satisfying snack.

Veggie Spring Rolls with Dipping Sauce

Ingredients:

- Rice paper wrappers
- Shredded lettuce
- Julienned carrots
- Sliced cucumber
- Sliced bell peppers
- Fresh mint leaves
- Fresh cilantro leaves
- Cooked and sliced shrimp or tofu (optional for protein)

Dipping Sauce:

- 1/4 cup low-sodium soy sauce
- 1 tablespoon rice vinegar
- 1 tablespoon honey
- 1/2 teaspoon grated ginger
- 1/2 teaspoon minced garlic
- 1/4 teaspoon sesame oil
- 1/4 teaspoon red pepper flakes (optional for spice)

Instructions:

1. Prepare a shallow dish filled with warm water to soften the rice paper wrappers.
2. Dip one rice paper wrapper into the warm water for a few seconds until it becomes pliable.
3. Place the softened wrapper on a clean work surface.
4. Layer the shredded lettuce, julienned carrots, sliced cucumber, sliced bell peppers, fresh mint leaves, fresh cilantro leaves, and cooked and sliced shrimp or tofu (if using) on the lower half of the rice paper wrapper.
5. Carefully fold the sides of the wrapper over the filling and roll it tightly into a spring roll shape.

6. Repeat the process with the remaining ingredients.

7. In a small bowl, whisk together the low-sodium soy sauce, rice vinegar, honey, grated ginger, minced garlic, sesame oil, and red pepper flakes (if using) to prepare the dipping sauce.

8. Serve the veggie spring rolls with the dipping sauce for a refreshing and nutrient-packed appetizer.

Chapter 6: Desserts

Desserts hold a special place in our hearts and taste buds, but for those on a kidney dialysis diet, finding delicious yet kidney-friendly options can be challenging. Fear not, as we have curated a delightful selection of desserts that will satisfy your sweet cravings without compromising your health.

Baked Apples with Cinnamon

Ingredients:

- 4 medium-sized apples (Granny Smith or Honeycrisp work well)
- 2 tablespoons unsalted butter, melted
- 1 tablespoon brown sugar (or a sugar substitute)
- 1 teaspoon ground cinnamon
- 1/4 cup chopped walnuts (optional)

Instructions:

1. Preheat your oven to 375°F (190°C).

2. Wash the apples thoroughly and core them, creating a cavity in the center to hold the filling.

3. In a small bowl, combine the melted butter, brown sugar, and ground cinnamon.

4. Brush the mixture over the inside and outside of the apples.

5. Place the apples in a baking dish and fill the centers with the remaining cinnamon-butter mixture.

6. Optionally, sprinkle chopped walnuts over the top for added crunch and flavor.

7. Bake in the preheated oven for about 25-30 minutes or until the apples are tender.

8. Serve warm, and if desired, drizzle with a touch of honey or a dollop of low-phosphorus whipped cream.

Banana and Strawberry Popsicles

Ingredients:

- 2 ripe bananas
- 1 cup fresh strawberries, hulled
- 1 cup plain Greek yogurt (low-phosphorus)
- 1 tablespoon honey (optional, for added sweetness)

Instructions:

1. In a blender, combine the ripe bananas, fresh strawberries, and Greek yogurt.
2. If you prefer a sweeter taste, add a tablespoon of honey to the mixture.
3. Blend until you have a smooth and creamy consistency.
4. Pour the mixture into popsicle molds or small paper cups.
5. Insert popsicle sticks into each mold.
6. Freeze the popsicles for at least 4-6 hours or until fully set.
7. To remove the popsicles from the molds, briefly dip them in warm water to loosen the edges.
8. Enjoy these refreshing and nutritious popsicles on a hot day!

Chocolate Chia Seed Pudding

Ingredients:

- 1/4 cup chia seeds
- 1 cup unsweetened almond milk (or any low-potassium milk substitute)

- 2 tablespoons unsweetened cocoa powder
- 1-2 tablespoons honey or maple syrup (optional, for sweetness)
- 1/2 teaspoon vanilla extract
- Fresh berries for topping

Instructions:

1. In a mixing bowl, combine the chia seeds, unsweetened almond milk, cocoa powder, honey (if using), and vanilla extract.
2. Mix well until all the ingredients are fully incorporated.
3. Cover the bowl and refrigerate the mixture for at least 2-4 hours, or ideally overnight. This will allow the chia seeds to absorb the liquid and form a pudding-like consistency.
4. Before serving, give the chia seed pudding a good stir to ensure a smooth texture.
5. Spoon the pudding into individual serving dishes and top with fresh berries for an extra burst of flavor and antioxidants.

Lemon Ricotta Cake (Low-Phosphorus)

Ingredients:

- 1 cup all-purpose flour
- 1/2 cup almond flour
- 1 teaspoon baking powder
- 1/4 teaspoon salt
- 1 cup ricotta cheese (low-phosphorus)
- 1/2 cup unsalted butter, softened
- 3/4 cup granulated sugar
- 2 large eggs
- Zest of 2 lemons
- Juice of 1 lemon
- 1 teaspoon vanilla extract
- Powdered sugar for dusting (optional)

Instructions:

1. Preheat your oven to 350°F (175°C) and grease a 9-inch round cake pan.
2. In a medium bowl, whisk together the all-purpose flour, almond flour, baking powder, and salt.

3. In a separate large bowl, beat the softened butter and granulated sugar until light and fluffy.

4. Add the eggs one at a time, beating well after each addition.

5. Stir in the ricotta cheese, lemon zest, lemon juice, and vanilla extract until well combined.

6. Gradually add the dry flour mixture to the wet ingredients, mixing until just combined.

7. Pour the batter into the prepared cake pan and smooth the top with a spatula.

8. Bake in the preheated oven for approximately 35-40 minutes or until a toothpick inserted into the center comes out clean.

9. Allow the cake to cool in the pan for about 10 minutes before transferring it to a wire rack to cool completely.

10. Dust the top of the cake with powdered sugar, if desired, before serving this delightful low-phosphorus lemon ricotta cake.

Vanilla Yogurt with Fresh Berries

Ingredients:

- 1 cup plain Greek yogurt (low-phosphorus)
- 1 teaspoon pure vanilla extract
- Fresh mixed berries (blueberries, strawberries, raspberries) for topping
- 1 tablespoon chopped almonds or walnuts (optional, for added crunch)

Instructions:

1. In a bowl, combine the plain Greek yogurt and vanilla extract.
2. Mix well until the vanilla is evenly distributed in the yogurt.
3. Spoon the vanilla yogurt into serving bowls or glasses.
4. Top with an assortment of fresh mixed berries and, if desired, a sprinkle of chopped almonds or walnuts for added texture.
5. Enjoy this simple yet nutritious dessert that's bursting with the natural sweetness of fresh berries!

Poached Pears in Red Wine

Ingredients:

- 4 ripe but firm pears (such as Bartlett or Bosc)
- 2 cups red wine (low in potassium)
- 1/2 cup water
- 1/2 cup granulated sugar
- 1 cinnamon stick
- 1 vanilla bean (split and scraped)
- Zest of 1 orange

Instructions:

1. Peel the pears, leaving the stems intact, and cut a small slice off the bottom of each pear to help them stand upright.
2. In a saucepan, combine the red wine, water, granulated sugar, cinnamon stick, vanilla bean, and orange zest.
3. Bring the mixture to a gentle simmer over medium heat, stirring occasionally to dissolve the sugar.
4. Add the peeled pears to the poaching liquid and reduce the heat to low.

5. Simmer the pears for about 15-20 minutes or until they are tender but not mushy, turning them occasionally to ensure even poaching.
6. Remove the saucepan from the heat and allow the pears to cool in the poaching liquid.
7. Once cooled, transfer the poached pears to individual serving dishes and drizzle with some of the red wine syrup from the poaching liquid.
8. Serve the poached pears with a dollop of low-phosphorus whipped cream or a scoop of low-potassium sorbet for an elegant and refreshing dessert.

Watermelon Sorbet (Low-Potassium)

Ingredients:

- 4 cups seedless watermelon, cubed
- 1/4 cup freshly squeezed lime juice
- 1/4 cup honey (or a sugar substitute)

Instructions:

1. In a blender, combine the cubed watermelon, freshly squeezed lime juice, and honey.

2. Blend until you have a smooth and homogeneous mixture.

3. Taste the sorbet mixture and adjust the sweetness to your preference by adding more honey if needed.

4. Pour the sorbet mixture into a shallow dish or a metal baking pan.

5. Place the dish in the freezer and let it freeze for about 2-3 hours or until the sorbet is firm but not too hard.

6. Once the sorbet is ready, use a fork to scrape the frozen mixture, creating a fluffy and icy texture.

7. Serve the watermelon sorbet in chilled bowls or glasses for a delightful low-potassium treat on a warm day!

Pineapple Coconut Ice Cream (Low-Sodium)

Ingredients:

- 2 cups fresh pineapple chunks

- 1 can (14 ounces) coconut milk (unsweetened)
- 2 tablespoons honey (or a sugar substitute)
- 1 teaspoon pure vanilla extract

Instructions:

1. In a blender, combine the fresh pineapple chunks, coconut milk, honey (or a sugar substitute), and vanilla extract.
2. Blend until you have a smooth and creamy mixture.
3. Taste the ice cream base and adjust the sweetness according to your preference.
4. Pour the mixture into an ice cream maker and churn it according to the manufacturer's instructions until it reaches a soft-serve consistency.
5. Transfer the churned ice cream into an airtight container and freeze it for an additional 2-3 hours to firm up.
6. Serve the delightful pineapple coconut ice cream in scoops or cones for a tropical escape, minus the sodium!

Berry Parfait with Whipped Cream

Ingredients:

- 1 cup low-phosphorus whipped cream (store-bought or homemade)
- 1 cup fresh mixed berries (blueberries, strawberries, raspberries)
- 1/2 cup granola (low-phosphorus)

Instructions:

1. In a glass or a parfait dish, layer the low-phosphorus whipped cream, fresh mixed berries, and granola.
2. Repeat the layers to create a visually appealing and delightful dessert.
3. Top the parfait with a few more fresh berries for garnish.
4. Enjoy the luscious berry parfait, a heavenly combination of creaminess, sweetness, and crunch!

Almond Flour Brownies

Ingredients:

- 1 cup almond flour

- 1/4 cup unsweetened cocoa powder
- 1/2 teaspoon baking soda
- 1/4 teaspoon salt
- 1/2 cup unsalted butter, melted
- 1/2 cup granulated sugar
- 1/4 cup honey (or a sugar substitute)
- 2 large eggs
- 1 teaspoon pure vanilla extract
- 1/2 cup dark chocolate chips (optional, for added indulgence)

Instructions:

1. Preheat your oven to 350°F (175°C) and grease an 8-inch square baking pan.
2. In a medium bowl, whisk together the almond flour, unsweetened cocoa powder, baking soda, and salt.
3. In a separate large bowl, mix the melted butter, granulated sugar, and honey until well combined.
4. Add the eggs one at a time, stirring well after each addition.
5. Stir in the pure vanilla extract.

6. Gradually add the dry flour mixture to the wet ingredients, mixing until just combined.

7. If desired, fold in the dark chocolate chips for added richness and decadence.

8. Pour the brownie batter into the prepared baking pan, spreading it out evenly.

9. Bake in the preheated oven for approximately 20-25 minutes or until a toothpick inserted into the center comes out with a few moist crumbs.

10. Allow the almond flour brownies to cool in the pan for a few minutes before cutting them into squares.

11. Serve the delightful almond flour brownies with a scoop of low-potassium ice cream or a dollop of low-phosphorus whipped cream for an indulgent treat without the guilt!

Chapter 7: Smoothies

In this chapter, we will explore ten unique and delectable smoothie recipes that cater to various dietary needs, including low-potassium, low-phosphorus, and low-sodium options.

Berry Blast Smoothie (Low-Potassium):

Ingredients:
- 1 cup of frozen mixed berries (strawberries, blueberries, raspberries)
- 1 ripe banana
- 1/2 cup of unsweetened almond milk
- 1 tablespoon of chia seeds
- 1 tablespoon of honey (optional for added sweetness)
- Ice cubes (optional, for a thicker consistency)

Instructions:

1. Peel and slice the banana, then add it to the blender along with the frozen mixed berries.
2. Pour in the unsweetened almond milk, ensuring it covers the fruits adequately.
3. For an extra boost of fiber and omega-3 fatty acids, sprinkle in the chia seeds.
4. For a touch of sweetness, drizzle honey into the mix (optional).
5. Blend all the ingredients until smooth and creamy, adding ice cubes if desired for a thicker texture.
6. Pour the Berry Blast Smoothie into a glass, and it's ready to serve. Enjoy the burst of berry goodness!

Green Goddess Smoothie:

Ingredients:
- 1 ripe avocado
- 1 cup of fresh spinach leaves
- 1/2 cup of diced cucumber
- 1/2 cup of green grapes
- 1 cup of coconut water
- 1 tablespoon of fresh lime juice
- Honey or agave syrup (optional, for sweetness)

Instructions:

1. Cut the avocado in half, remove the pit, and scoop out the flesh into the blender.
2. Add the fresh spinach leaves and diced cucumber to the mix.
3. Toss in the green grapes for a burst of natural sweetness.
4. Pour in the refreshing coconut water, followed by a tablespoon of lime juice for a tangy twist.
5. If you prefer a sweeter taste, add a drizzle of honey or agave syrup (optional).
6. Blend all the ingredients until smooth and velvety green.
7. Pour the Green Goddess Smoothie into a tall glass, and it's ready to refresh your senses!

Tropical Mango-Pineapple Smoothie:

Ingredients:

- 1 ripe mango, peeled and pitted
- 1 cup of fresh pineapple chunks

- 1/2 cup of coconut milk
- 1/2 cup of orange juice
- 1 tablespoon of shredded coconut (optional, for garnish)
- Mint leaves (optional, for garnish)

Instructions:

1. Slice the ripe mango and remove the pit, then add the mango chunks to the blender.
2. Toss in the fresh pineapple chunks for a tropical twist.
3. Pour in the creamy coconut milk and tangy orange juice to enhance the flavors.
4. For an exotic touch, sprinkle shredded coconut on top (optional).
5. Blend all the ingredients until smooth and lusciously tropical.
6. Garnish the Tropical Mango-Pineapple Smoothie with a few fresh mint leaves.
7. Pour the refreshing blend into a chilled glass, and it's time to savor the taste of the tropics!

Creamy Avocado Smoothie:

Ingredients:

- 1 ripe avocado
- 1 ripe banana
- 1 cup of unsweetened almond milk
- 1 tablespoon of almond butter
- 1 tablespoon of honey (optional, for sweetness)
- Ice cubes (optional, for a chilled texture)

Instructions:

1. Scoop out the creamy flesh of the ripe avocado and place it in the blender.
2. Add the ripe banana to the mix for natural sweetness and a smoother texture.
3. Pour in the unsweetened almond milk, followed by a tablespoon of almond butter for richness.
4. For an extra touch of sweetness, drizzle honey into the mix (optional).
5. If you prefer a chilled smoothie, add some ice cubes before blending.
6. Blend all the ingredients until the Creamy Avocado Smoothie is velvety and luscious.

7. Pour the smoothie into a tall glass, and it's ready to satisfy your taste buds with its creamy goodness!

Spinach and Banana Smoothie (Low-Phosphorus):

Ingredients:
- 1 ripe banana
- 1 cup of fresh spinach leaves
- 1/2 cup of unsweetened almond milk
- 1 tablespoon of ground flaxseed
- 1 tablespoon of honey (optional, for added sweetness)
- Ice cubes (optional, for a chilled texture)

Instructions:
1. Peel and slice the ripe banana, then add it to the blender.
2. Add the fresh spinach leaves to the mix for a boost of nutrients.
3. Pour in the unsweetened almond milk for a creamy base.

4. For an extra dose of omega-3 fatty acids, sprinkle in the ground flaxseed.

5. If you prefer a sweeter smoothie, drizzle honey into the mix (optional).

6. For a chilled delight, add some ice cubes before blending.

7. Blend all the ingredients until the Spinach and Banana Smoothie is smooth and vibrant.

8. Pour the nutritious smoothie into a glass, and it's ready to energize your day!

Cherry-Almond Smoothie (Low-Sodium):

Ingredients:
- 1 cup of frozen cherries
- 1 ripe banana
- 1 cup of unsweetened almond milk
- 1 tablespoon of almond butter
- 1 teaspoon of vanilla extract
- Ice cubes (optional, for a cooler texture)

Instructions:

1. Add the frozen cherries to the blender for a burst of sweet-tart flavor.

2. Peel and slice the ripe banana, then add it to the mix for natural sweetness.

3. Pour in the unsweetened almond milk, followed by a tablespoon of almond butter for creaminess.

4. Add a teaspoon of vanilla extract for a delightful aroma.

5. For a cooler Cherry-Almond Smoothie, toss in some ice cubes before blending.

6. Blend all the ingredients until the smoothie is creamy and enticingly pink.

7. Pour the Cherry-Almond Smoothie into a chilled glass, and it's ready to relish!

Orange Creamsicle Smoothie:

Ingredients:

- 1 large orange, peeled and segmented
- 1/2 cup of Greek yogurt (plain or vanilla-flavored)
- 1/2 cup of unsweetened almond milk

- 1 tablespoon of honey (optional, for added sweetness)
- 1 teaspoon of vanilla extract
- Ice cubes (optional, for a cooler texture)

Instructions:

1. Peel and segment the large orange, then add the juicy segments to the blender.
2. Add the creamy Greek yogurt to the mix for a tangy twist.
3. Pour in the unsweetened almond milk, followed by a teaspoon of vanilla extract for that classic creamsicle taste.
4. For an extra touch of sweetness, drizzle honey into the mix (optional).
5. For a cooler and creamier Orange Creamsicle Smoothie, add some ice cubes before blending.
6. Blend all the ingredients until the smoothie is creamy and citrusy.
7. Pour the delightful Orange Creamsicle Smoothie into a tall glass, and it's ready to transport you to a nostalgic treat!

Cucumber and Mint Smoothie:

Ingredients:

- 1 medium cucumber, peeled and chopped
- 1 cup of fresh spinach leaves
- 1/2 cup of fresh mint leaves
- 1/2 cup of plain Greek yogurt
- 1 tablespoon of honey (optional, for added sweetness)
- 1 tablespoon of fresh lime juice
- Ice cubes (optional, for a refreshing texture)

Instructions:

1. Peel and chop the medium cucumber, then add it to the blender.
2. Toss in the fresh spinach leaves and mint leaves for a rejuvenating green blend.
3. Add the creamy plain Greek yogurt to the mix for a smooth texture.
4. Pour in the fresh lime juice for a zesty kick.
5. For an extra touch of sweetness, drizzle honey into the mix (optional).

6. For a refreshing and cooler Cucumber and Mint Smoothie, add some ice cubes before blending.

7. Blend all the ingredients until the smoothie is refreshing and packed with green goodness.

8. Pour the revitalizing Cucumber and Mint Smoothie into a chilled glass, and it's ready to invigorate your senses!

Kiwi-Strawberry Smoothie:

Ingredients:

- 2 ripe kiwis, peeled and diced
- 1 cup of fresh strawberries, hulled
- 1/2 cup of coconut water
- 1/2 cup of plain Greek yogurt
- 1 tablespoon of honey (optional, for added sweetness)
- Ice cubes (optional, for a cooler texture)

Instructions:

1. Peel and dice the ripe kiwis, then add them to the blender.

2. Add the fresh strawberries to the mix for a burst of sweetness and vibrant color.

3. Pour in the hydrating coconut water, followed by the creamy plain Greek yogurt for a smooth consistency.

4. For an extra touch of sweetness, drizzle honey into the mix (optional).

5. For a cooler and creamier Kiwi-Strawberry Smoothie, add some ice cubes before blending.

6. Blend all the ingredients until the smoothie is refreshingly pink and deliciously fruity.

7. Pour the tropical Kiwi-Strawberry Smoothie into a tall glass, and it's ready to brighten up your day!

Peach and Greek Yogurt Smoothie:

Ingredients:

- 2 ripe peaches, peeled and pitted
- 1/2 cup of plain Greek yogurt
- 1/2 cup of unsweetened almond milk
- 1 tablespoon of honey (optional, for added sweetness)
- 1 teaspoon of vanilla extract

- Ice cubes (optional, for a cooler texture)

Instructions:

1. Peel and pit the ripe peaches, then chop them and add them to the blender.
2. Add the creamy plain Greek yogurt to the mix for a protein-packed base.
3. Pour in the unsweetened almond milk, followed by a teaspoon of vanilla extract for a delightful aroma.
4. For an extra touch of sweetness, drizzle honey into the mix (optional).
5. For a cooler and creamier Peach and Greek Yogurt Smoothie, add some ice cubes before blending.
6. Blend all the ingredients until the smoothie is creamy and peachy.
7. Pour the luscious Peach and Greek Yogurt Smoothie into a chilled glass, and it's ready to treat your taste buds!

CONCLUSION

As we reach the end of this comprehensive guide on the Kidney Dialysis Diet for beginners, we come to a crucial section - the conclusion. Throughout this journey, we have delved into the importance of understanding and following a kidney-friendly diet to maintain optimal health while undergoing dialysis treatment. Let's recap some key points and explore a deeper understanding of how you can continue on your path to kidney wellness.

Embracing a Lifestyle of Wellness

In conclusion, it is essential to emphasize that the kidney dialysis diet is not just a temporary regimen but a way of life. Adopting a kidney-friendly lifestyle will not only positively impact your physical health but also your overall well-being. Embrace this journey with optimism and determination, knowing that you are taking vital steps towards a healthier and happier life.

Maintaining a Healthy Kidney Dialysis Diet

As we've learned, the kidney dialysis diet aims to manage and control certain nutrients, such as potassium, phosphorus, sodium, and protein, to alleviate the burden on your kidneys. It is crucial to continue monitoring your food choices, portion sizes, and nutrient intake to maintain the proper balance. Consulting with a registered dietitian will prove valuable in crafting personalized meal plans tailored to your specific needs.

Creating Your Personalized Meal Plans

Every individual is unique, and so are their dietary requirements. While this guide offers a 30-day meal plan, it is essential to create a personalized approach based on your medical history, lab results, and preferences. Work closely with your healthcare team, especially a registered dietitian or nutritionist, to develop a meal plan that suits your lifestyle and health goals.

Tips for Dining Out on a Dialysis Diet

Eating out at restaurants or social gatherings can be challenging while following a kidney dialysis diet. However, with the right knowledge and planning, it can be an enjoyable experience. When dining out, communicate your dietary restrictions to the server and inquire about suitable options. Choose dishes that align with your diet goals and consider making simple modifications if needed.

Staying Hydrated and Active for Kidney Health

Proper hydration is fundamental for kidney health. Always ensure you drink an adequate amount of water each day unless advised otherwise by your healthcare team due to specific medical conditions. Regular physical activity is also crucial for overall well-being. Engage in activities that you enjoy and are approved by your healthcare provider. Staying active can improve circulation, strengthen muscles, and support kidney function.

www.ingramcontent.com/pod-product-compliance
Lightning Source LLC
Chambersburg PA
CBHW062339290526
45794CB00005B/2060